Fatma Chaker
Mohamed Derbel
Fatma Khanfir

Why do women shy away from elective C-sections?

Fatma Chaker
Mohamed Derbel
Fatma Khanfir

Why do women shy away from elective C-sections?

ScienciaScripts

Imprint

Cover image: www.ingimage.com

This book is a translation from the original published under ISBN 978-620-6-71529-0.

Publisher:
Sciencia Scripts
is a trademark of
Dodo Books Indian Ocean Ltd. and OmniScriptum S.R.L publishing group

120 High Road, East Finchley, London, N2 9ED, United Kingdom
Str. Armeneasca 28/1, office 1, Chisinau MD-2012, Republic of Moldova, Europe
Managing Directors: Ieva Konstantinova, Victoria Ursu
info@omniscriptum.com

Printed at: see last page
ISBN: 978-620-8-55524-5

Contents

1 INTRODUCTION

In the collective imagination, pregnancy and childbirth are often perceived as moments of joy. However, from a scientific point of view, pregnancy is a period of major transition for women, marked by considerable emotional changes and physiological, biological and psychological alterations likely to have an impact on their mental health (Dimassi et al., 2021).

Throughout the centuries, the pain of childbirth has been a major preoccupation for women, giving rise to numerous investigations. Today, thanks to advances in epidural analgesia techniques, the sensation of pain during labour has been considerably reduced. In France, the majority of women opt for this method of analgesia. However, despite this possibility of pain management, childbirth remains an event fraught with anxiety for most women. It is associated with deep-seated apprehensions, influenced by personal, family and cultural factors, and continues to be a crucial moment in the lives of women and couples (Leclerc, 1993).

In the general population, around 80% of women express fear at the thought of giving birth. Excessive and persistent fear of childbirth is known as tocophobia, a little-known anxiety disorder characterised by avoidance behaviour during pregnancy that can have significant emotional and physical repercussions. This phobia of childbirth seems to be relatively common, affecting more than 20% of pregnant women in a mild to moderate way, and between 6 and 11% in a severe and disabling way. In the most serious cases, this can lead the mother-to-be to request a caesarean section without any medical reason, which can be worrying. (Riquet et al., 2020)

In recent years, according to the WHO, the caesarean section rate has increased remarkably worldwide, ranging from 1% to 58% (Dumont & Guilmoto, 2020).

Similarly, in Tunisia, the caesarean section rate has reached 50% of all births recorded since 2021 (Zouaoui, 2021).

In a statement made on the fringes of the annual Gynaecology and Obstetrics conference, it was pointed out that Caesarean section deliveries have risen steadily from one year to the next, with the rate not exceeding 11% during the 1990s (Riquet et al., 2020).

It should be noted that in Tunisia, women are not involved in decision-making about their childbirth. We do not currently have any data that would enable us to
to shed light on their thoughts, fears and desired mode of delivery (Dimassi et al., 2021). To this end, we carried out this study with the aim of analysing the opinion of a sample of Tunisian women concerning the right to free choice of the route of their childbirth and determining the factors that could influence the route of childbirth. Chosen by the women.

Women may choose caesarean section for a variety of reasons, including medical complications, concerns about the safety of the baby or the mother, previous difficult labour experiences, personal factors such as fear of the pain associated with vaginal birth, or even fear of the impact of vaginal birth on their sex life.

All pregnant women feel a little anxious about the approach of childbirth. However, around 20% of women dare to say that they are afraid of giving birth, and 6-10% suffer from outright tocophobia (Lucie & Chagno, 2009).

This work is divided into several parts. Firstly, it presents the problem, the aim and the question of our research. The second part describes the methodology used. The third part is devoted to the results obtained from the statistical analyses, as well as a discussion that feeds

into the interpretation of the results.
The conclusion provides us with an opportunity to present some solutions for reducing the caesarean section rate and to explain the importance of preparation for birth and parenthood (PNP) in achieving this objective.

The objectives of our work were:

1- Describe women's knowledge of vaginal birth.

2- To explore the factors associated with escape from vaginal delivery.

3-Describe the level of fear of vaginal delivery (by EPA: fear of childbirth scale) and its correlation with flight to caesarean delivery.

2 MATERIALS AND METHODS

1. MATERIAL

1.1. Type of study

This was a descriptive and analytical cross-sectional study, conducted from 15 January 2024 to 15 March 2024 at the CHU Hedi Chaker Sfax. Recruitment took place at the outpatient clinic and the ultrasound room of the obstetrics and gynaecology department and the emergency room of the Hedi Chaker University Hospital in Sfax.

1.2. Study population

The target population was Tunisian women in their 2nd and 3rd trimesters.

The source population was Tunisian women in their 2nd and 3rd trimesters who visited the outpatient clinic and the ultrasound room of the obstetrics and gynaecology department and the emergency room of the Hedi Chaker University Hospital in Sfax.

We established inclusion and non-inclusion criteria.

1.2.1. Inclusion criteria

Our study included :

- Pregnant women in their 2nd and 3rd trimesters
- Women with obstetric conditions favourable to vaginal delivery.

1.2.2. Non-inclusion criteria

We did not include :

- Women in labour. Labour is defined as the combination of close and regular uterine contractions (UC), the frequency and duration of which increase progressively with changes in the cervix.
- Deaf-mute women.
- Women with a psychiatric history.
- Women with high-risk pregnancies.
- Women with a medical condition contraindicating vaginal delivery.

1.2.3. Sample size

The number of subjects required (n) was calculated using the following formula:

$$n = \frac{z^2 p(1-p)}{e^2}$$

(Z =1.96, e: precision (e max =0.05), p: prevalence)

This formula was applied taking into account the prevalence of caesarean section in Tunisia, which was estimated to be around 50% (Faten et al., 2017)

The number of subjects required was calculated to be around 380.

However, given the time constraints and the difficulty of recruitment, we limited the number of subjects to 200 women.

1.3. Instruments used

We conducted an interview, the average length of which was 10 minutes, and the language of communication was Arabic and/or French. We drew up a data collection form for (Appendix A), identifying :

1.3.1. Socio-demographic data and background.

- Age.
- Marital status.
- Geographical origin.
- Level of study.
- The work situation.
- Socio-economic level
- Personal medical and surgical history.
- Recent bereavement
- Sports activity

1.3.2. Gynaecological and obstetrical history

- Parity.
- Previous abortion (AVT)

Women who had given birth at least once were asked about their previous births:

- The mode and conditions of delivery: the term of delivery, the place of delivery, the use of episiotomy, informing the woman about the procedure.
- The notion of a negative experience of childbirth, defined by the existence of at least one of these conditions: Fetal death in utero (FIDU) or neonatal death, instrumental delivery, post partum haemorrhage (PPH) with or without a stay in an intensive care unit, retention of the last head and an infectious or thromboembolic post partum complication (PPC). These conditions were verified in the birth records.

1.3.3. Details of current pregnancy

- Gestational age at the time of the questionnaire.
- The notion of infertility.
- Whether or not the pregnancy was planned.
- Whether or not the baby's sex is desired.
- Pregnancy monitoring: a well-monitored pregnancy is defined by at least five prenatal consultations and three ultrasounds.
- Pathologies that appear during pregnancy.

1.3.4. Information received about labour and birth

- Addressing the subject of childbirth
- Sources of information on childbirth and labour
- Knowledge of ways to reduce pain
- Knowledge of epidural analgesia
- Knowledge of PNP preparation
- The choice of delivery route
- Reasons given by women for their choice of delivery route

1.3.5. Fear of Childbirth Scale (EPA)

For a detailed assessment of fear of childbirth, we opted for the Fear of Childbirth Scale (EPA) (Appendix B). It was constructed on the basis of the DSM IV-TR diagnostic criteria for post-traumatic stress disorder applied to an anticipated event, which also makes it possible to assess the criteria for specific phobia of childbirth. The EPA is adapted from the TES (Traumatic Event Scale). We have translated this scale into Arabic (Appendix C). It is composed of five factors (Riquet et al., 2020):

- F1: Anticipation of trauma: this is the mother's fear of something bad happening to her and her child (dying or being injured), with a feeling of anxiety and powerlessness.
- F2: Cognitive intrusions: are defined by unpleasant thoughts, dreams and images about

childbirth that invade the pregnant woman and cause her physical and psychological distress.

- F3: Avoidance: this is a collection of memories, thoughts and situations relating to pregnancy and childbirth which cause feelings of distress.
- F4: Blunting: defined by a persistent inability to feel positive emotions, a negative emotional state and a marked reduction in interest in important activities.
- F5: Hyperstimulation: marked by irritability and fits of anger, persistent exaggerated startle reactions, difficulty concentrating and difficulty falling asleep.

In total, the EPA comprises 21 items rated on a 4-point Likert scale from "not at all" to "often". The scores range from 21 to 84 points.

This scale has no cut-off point. The higher the score, the greater the level of fear.

2. ETHICAL CONSIDERATIONS

Confidentiality was ensured during data collection, and the forms were filled in anonymously. The questionnaire was confidential and anonymous in order to protect the privacy of the participants and to ensure that they were properly involved in the questionnaire. Consent was completely free and informed.

3. DATA ENTRY AND ANALYSIS

The completed forms were entered into SPSS (Statistical Package for the Social Sciences) version 20.

Quantitative variables were expressed as estimated means with standard deviations and minimum and maximum values.

Qualitative variables were expressed as numbers and percentages.

The univariate analytical study used the ANOVA test to compare the means between 2 groups. The Chi-2 test was used to compare categorical variables.

The significance level was set at 5%. Differences were considered significant for $p < 0.05$.

3 RESULTS

1. DESCRIPTIVE STUDY

During our study period, we enrolled 200 women who met the inclusion criteria.

1.1. Socio-demographic data and background.

1.1.1. Age

The average age of the women surveyed was 28.3 years, with a standard deviation of 5.7 [18-44 years] (Figure 1).

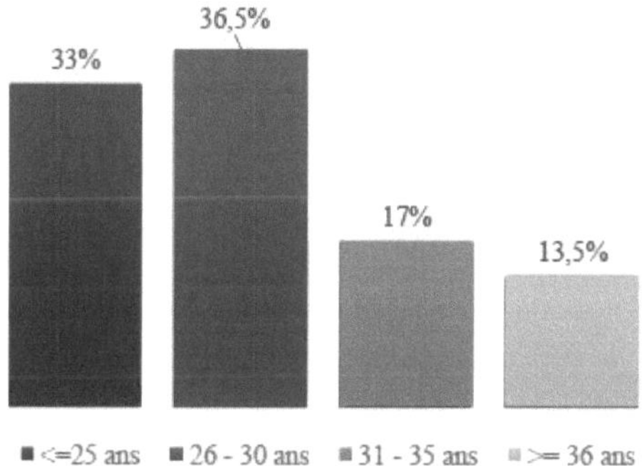

Figure 1: Breakdown of women by age

1.1.2. Marital status

Married women accounted for 97% of cases (Figure 2).

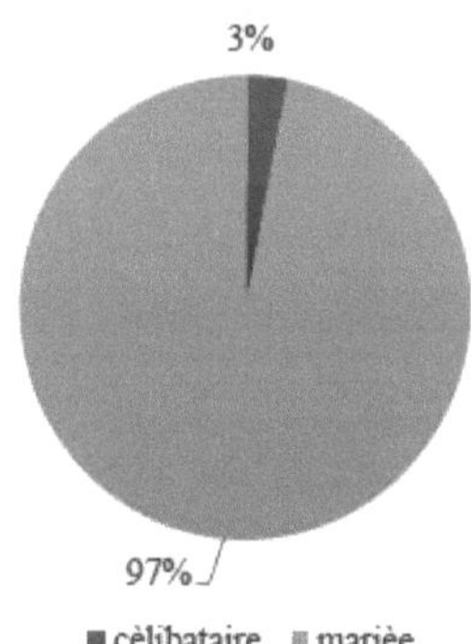

Figure 2: Breakdown of women by marital status

1.1.3. Geographical origin

In our study, 62% of the women were of urban origin (Figure 3).

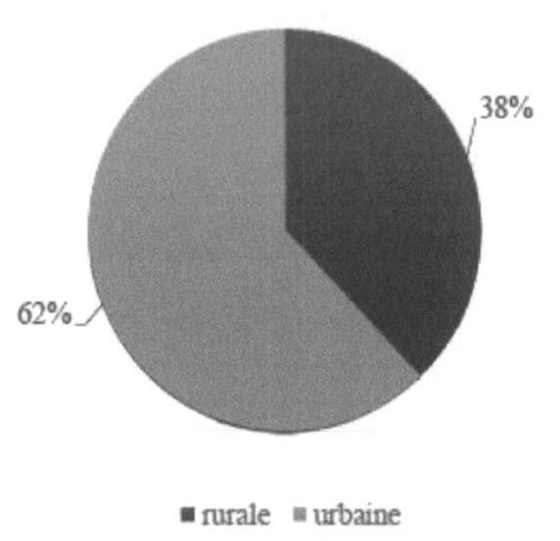

Figure 3: Breakdown of women by geographical origin

1.1.4. Level of study

In our population, 139 women (69.5%) had no more than secondary education (Figure 4).

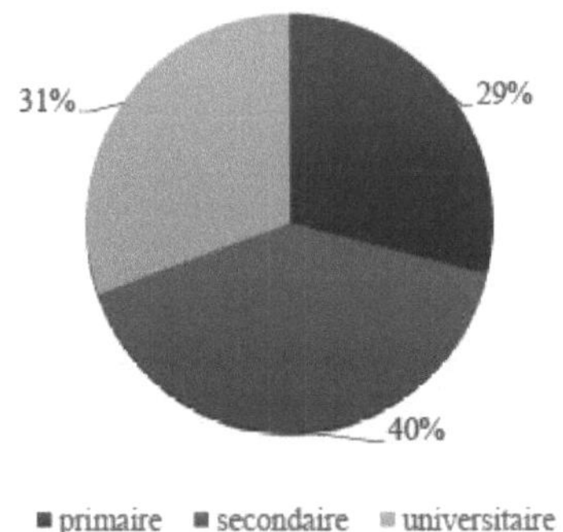

Figure 4: Breakdown of women by level of education

1.1.5. Professional situation

Housewife status was described for 159 women (79.5%) (Table I).

Table I: Breakdown of women by profession

	Workforce	Percentage
Housewife	159	**79,5%**
Civil servant	24	**12%**
Office functions	8	**4%**
Healthcare staff	5	**2,5%**
Worker	3	**1,5%**
Artisan	1	**0,5%**
Total	200	**100%**

1.1.6. Socio-economic level

The socio-economic level of the population was average for 85% of the women (Figure 5).

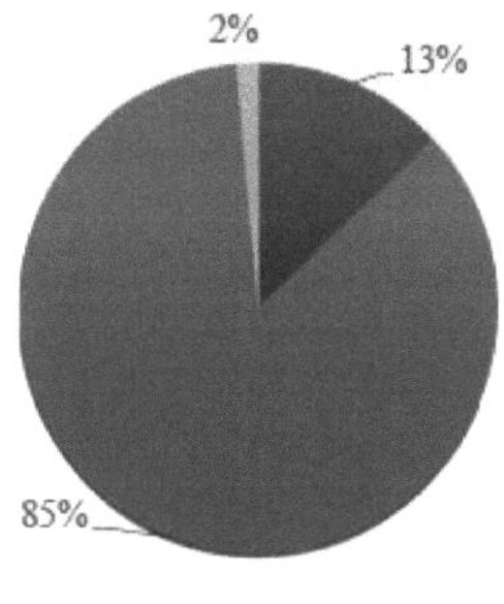

Figure 5: Breakdown of women by socio-economic level

1.1.7. Medical and surgical history

Medical history was reported in 58 women (29%) (Table II).

Table II: Women's medical history

Medical history	Number	Percentage
Anemia	31	15,5%
Diabetes	15	7,5%
Asthma	11	5,5%
Thrombocytopenia	3	1.5%
Thyroid	3	1,5%
Epilepsy	2	1%
Arterial hypertension (AH)	1	0,5%

A history of surgery was reported in 81 women (40.5%) (Table III).

Table III: Women's surgical history

Surgical history	Number	Percentage
Caesarean section	44	22%
Appendectomy	23	11,5%
Tonsillectomy	10	5%
Operated extra uterine pregnancy (EUP)	8	4%
Cholecystectomy	6	3%
Synechia repair	1	0,5%

It should be noted that one or more antecedents may be reported by a single patient.

1.2. Gynaeco-obstetrical history

1.2.1. Parity

In our study, 97 women (48.5%) were primiparous (Figure 6).

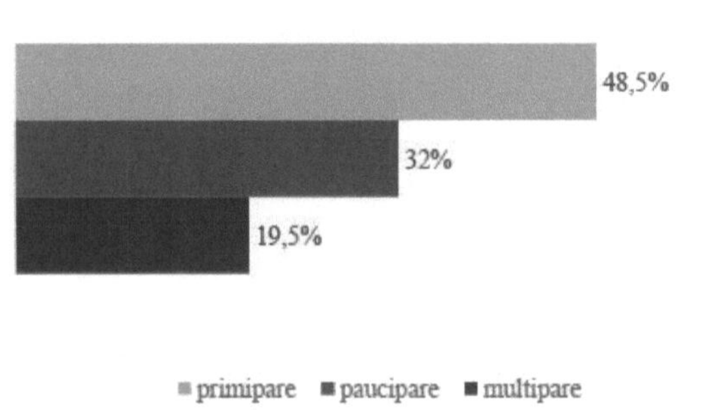

Figure 6: Breakdown of women by parity

1.2.2. History of abortion

In our series, a history of abortion was observed in 64 women (32%), 16 of whom (8%) had repeated abortions (Figure 7).

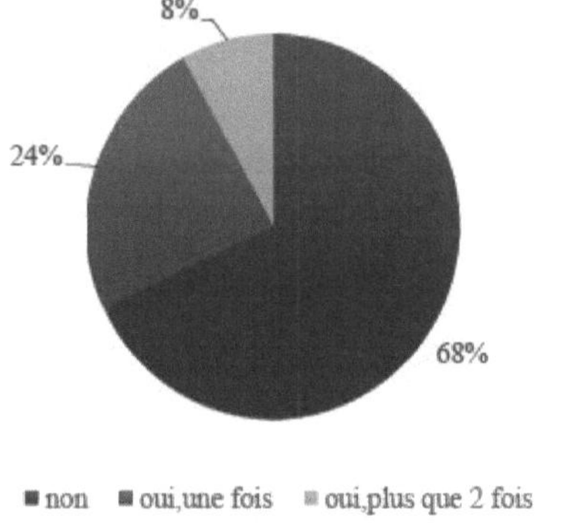

Figure 7: Breakdown of women by abortion history

1.3. Data relating to events and lifestyle

1.3.1. Recent bereavement

It was reported in 15 women (7.5%) (Figure 8).

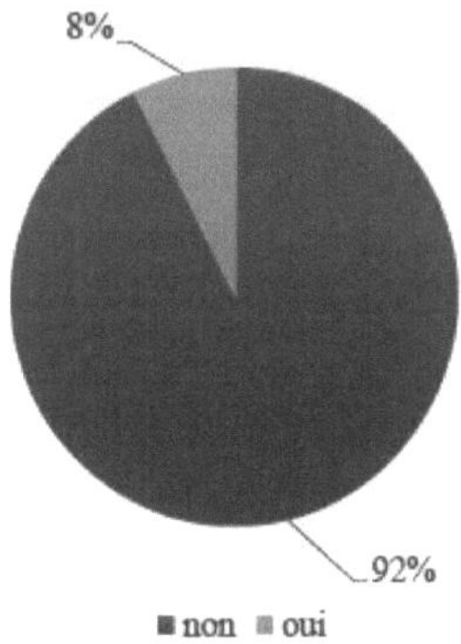

Figure 8: Breakdown of women by recent bereavement

1.3.2. Sporting activity

In our series, 27 women (13.5%) practised a sporting activity during pregnancy. In all cases, this sporting activity was represented by walking (Figure 9).

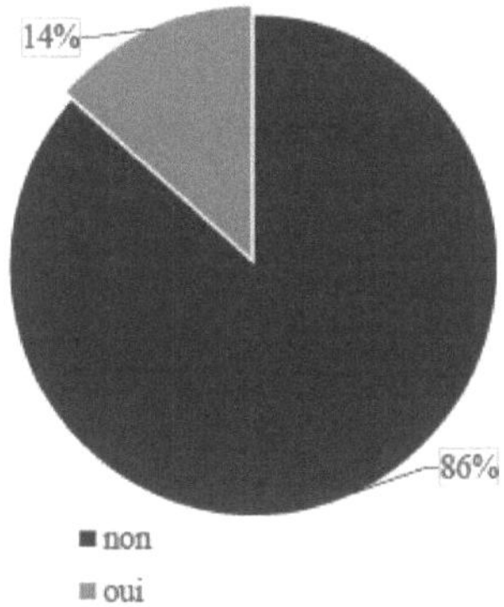

Figure 9: Breakdown of women by sporting activity

1.4. Data on previous deliveries

1.4.1. Term of delivery

Full-term deliveries were achieved by 94 women (90.4%) (Figure 10).

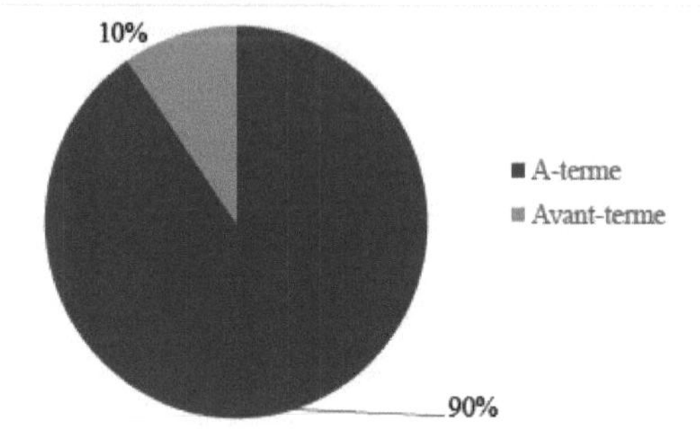

Figure 10: Breakdown of women by delivery date

1.4.2. Place of delivery

In our series, 83 women (79.8%) had given birth in a public hospital (Figure 11).

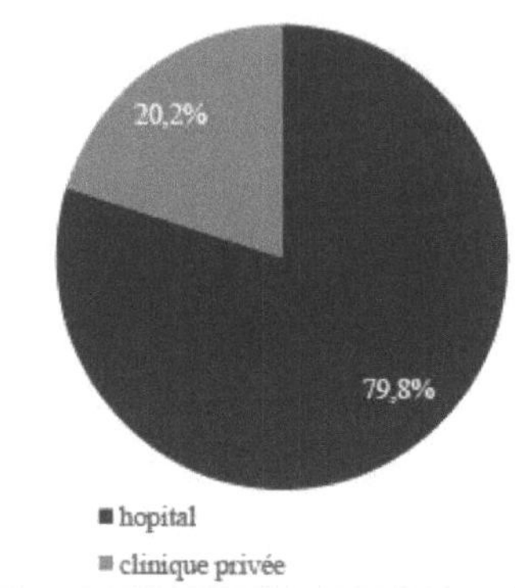

Figure 11: Breakdown of women by place of birth

1.4.3. Use of episiotomy

Episiotomy was performed in 55 women (52.9%), of whom 28 women (27.5%) were informed beforehand of the procedure (Figure 12).

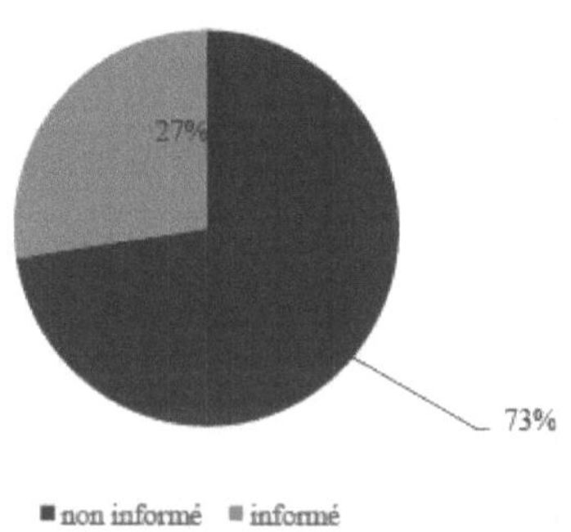

Figure 12: Distribution of women according to information prior to episiotomy

1.4.4. Negative experiences of childbirth

In 51.5% of women (n=103) who had given birth at least once, 77 women (79.3%) reported a negative experience (Table IV).

Table IV: Breakdown of women according to different negative experiences

	Number	Percentage
Instrumental delivery	20	15,4%
Fetal death in utero (FDIU)	17	13%
Neonatal death	13	10%
Post-partum haemorrhage (PPH)	12	9,2%
Breast complication	9	7%
Episiotomy infection	6	4,6%
Total	77	59,2%

It should be noted that one or more complications may be reported by a single patient.

1.5. Data relating to the current pregnancy

1.5.1. Gestational age at the time of the questionnaire

The mean gestational age was 34.72 SA with a standard deviation of 4.48 [16-41 SA] (Figure 13).

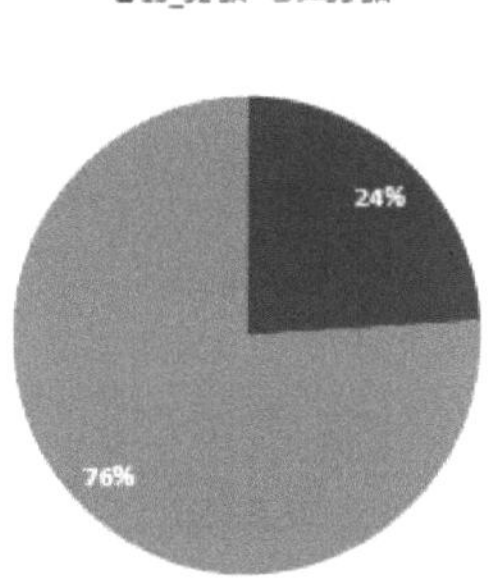

Figure 13: Distribution of women by gestational age at the time of the questionnaire

1.5.2. Concept of infertility

A history of infertility was noted in 27 women (13.5%) (Figure 14).

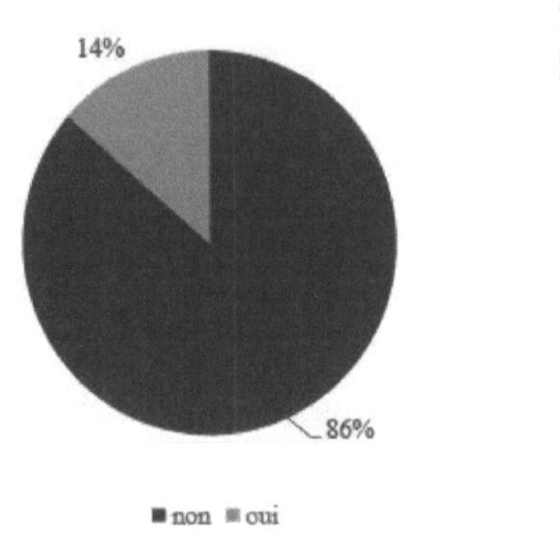

Figure 14: Breakdown of women with a history of infertility

Pregnancies were induced in 17 women (8.5%) (Figure 15).

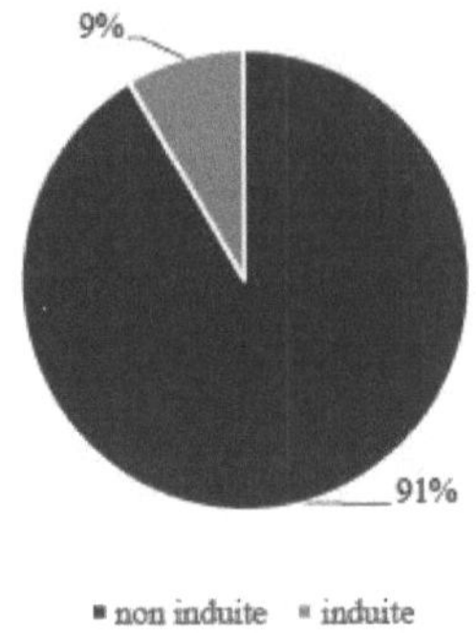

Figure 15: Distribution of women who have an induced pregnancy

1.5.3. Programming pregnancy

In our series, 141 pregnancies (70.5%) were planned (Figure 16).

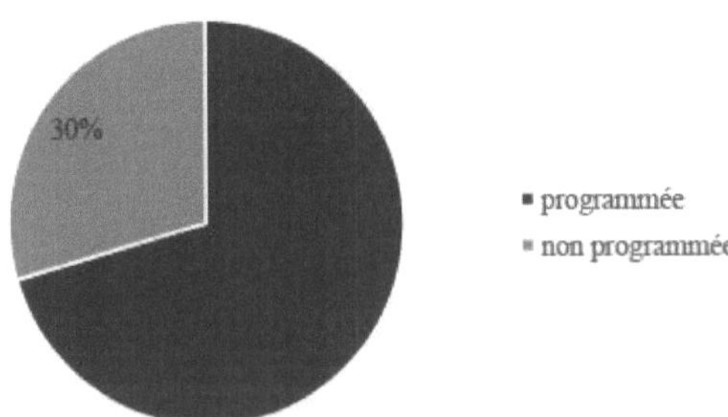

Figure 16: Distribution of women according to pregnancy planning

1.5.4. Pregnancy follow-up

Pregnancy was well monitored in 168 women (81%) (Figure 17).

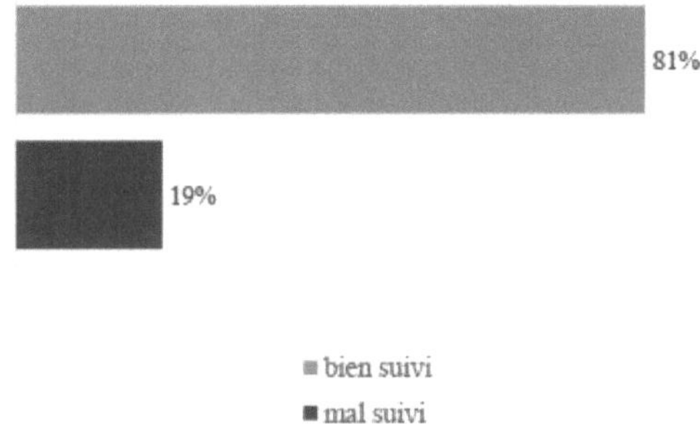

Figure 17: Breakdown of women by pregnancy status

17.5.5. Reaction to the baby's sex

In our series, 111 women (55.5%) wanted the sex of their babies (Figure 18).

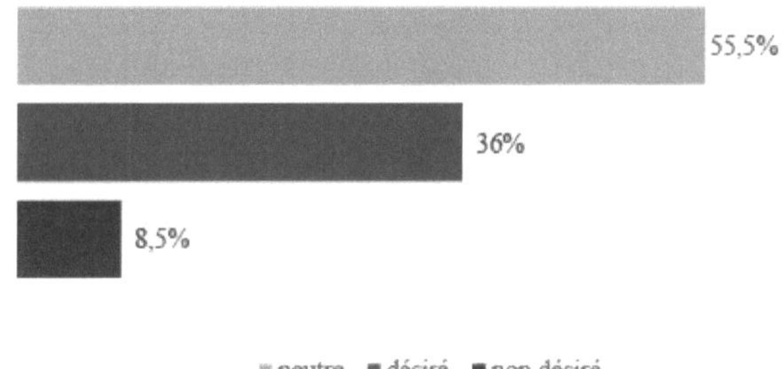

Figure 18: Distribution of women according to their desire for the sex of their baby

1.5.6. Somatic pathologies that appeared during pregnancy

In our series, 134 women (67%) had no somatic pathologies that appeared during pregnancy (Figure 19).

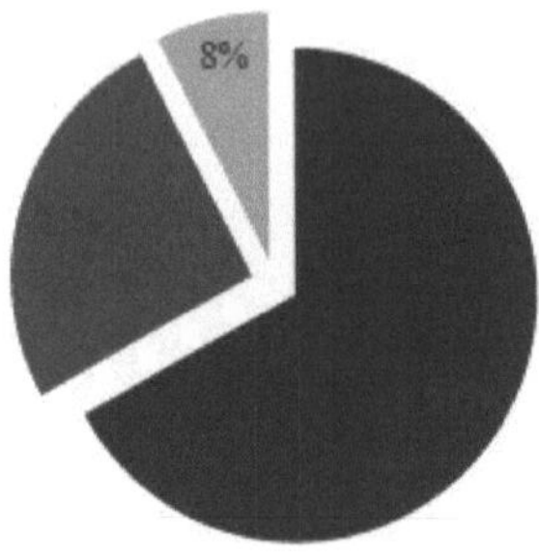

Figure 19: Breakdown of women by somatic complications

1.6. Women's knowledge of childbirth

1.6.1. Information received about labour and birth

In our series, 119 women (59.5%) were informed of the progress of labour and delivery. There were many sources of information (Table V).

Table V: Breakdown of women by source of information received

Source of information	Number	Percentage
Surroundings	162	81%
Internet, Forum	93	46,5%
Midwife	60	30%
Doctor	45	22,5%
Emissions	15	7,5%
Magazines, newspapers	14	7%

It should be noted that one or more reasons may be reported by a single patient.

1.6.2. Sources of concern for women

In our study, we found that 107 women (53.5%) had excessive fears about their baby's health (Figure 20).

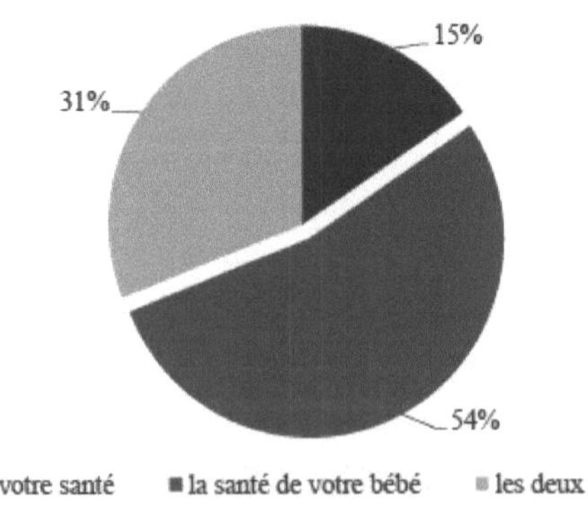

Figure 20: Breakdown of women by health concern

Of the 200 women surveyed, the birth itself was the most worrying phase of childbirth (Figure 21).

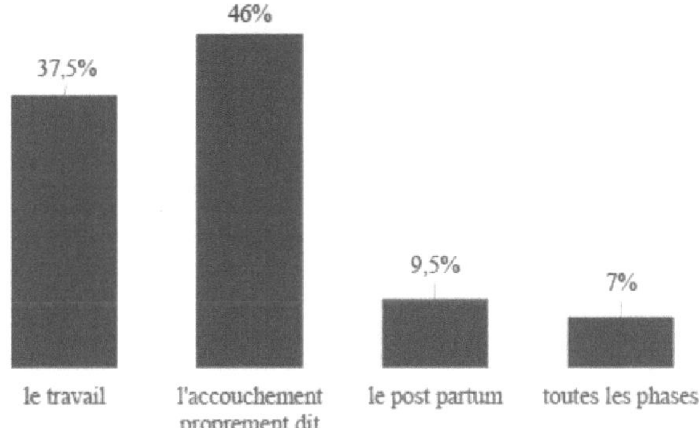

Figure 21: Breakdown of women by level of concern about the birth process

1.6.3. Women's knowledge of preparation for birth and parenthood, epidural analgesia and pain reduction:

Not all the women we interviewed had attended birth preparation classes during their pregnancies and 62% of women did not know what a PNP was. (Figure 22)

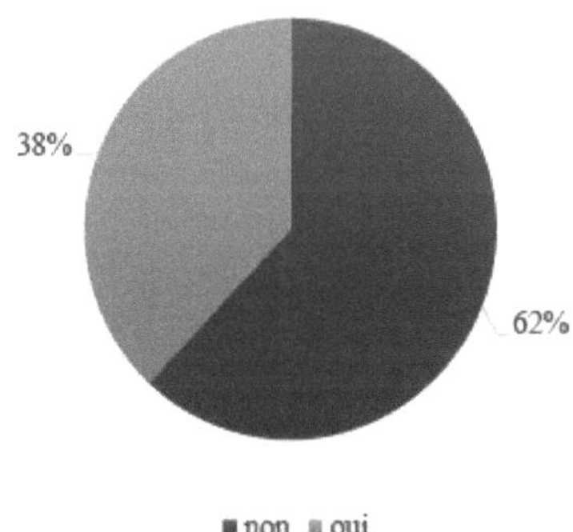

Figure 22: Distribution of women by knowledge of preparation for birth and parenthood and parenthood

We noted that 57% of women did not consider the epidural to be an effective treatment. method of reducing pain during vaginal delivery (Figure 23)

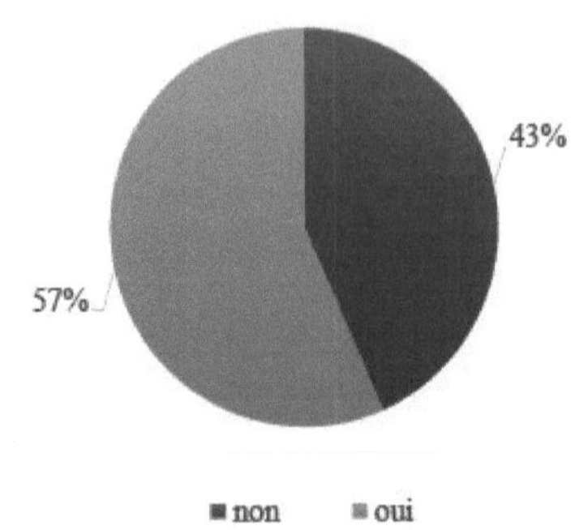

Figure 23: ***Breakdown of women by awareness of epidural***

In our series 162 (82%) women did not know how to reduce their pain (Figure 24).

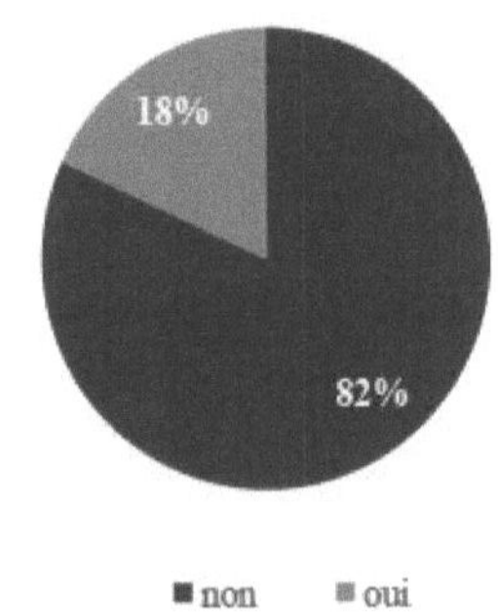

Figure 24: Breakdown of women by pain management

24.6.4. Choice of delivery route

In our study, 65.5% of women (n=131) chose to give birth by caesarean section if they had the choice. (Figure 25)

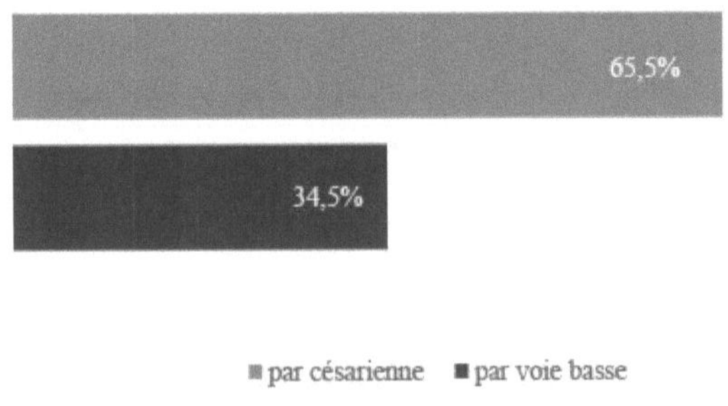

Figure 25: Breakdown of women by choice of delivery

25.6.4.1. Reasons for choosing Caesarean section

It should be noted that one or more reasons may be reported by a single patient (Figure 26).

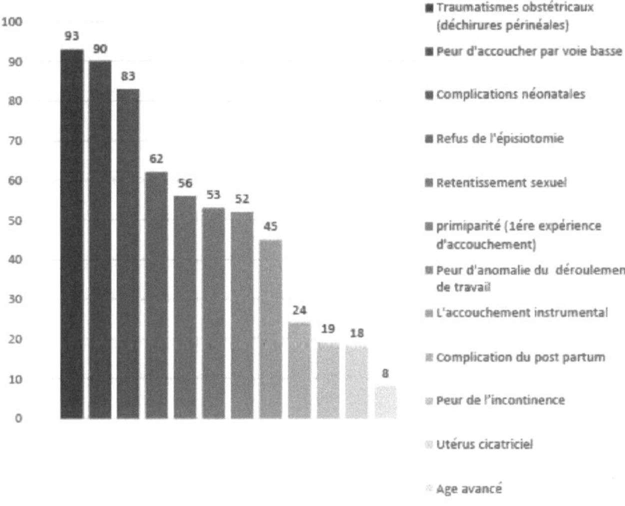

- Obstetric trauma (perineal tears)
- Fear of giving birth vaginally
- Neonatal complications
- Refusal of episiotomy
- Sexual repercussions
- primiparity (1st experience of childbirth)
- Fear of workflow anomalies
- Instrumental delivery
- Post partum complications
- Fear of incontinence
- Scarred uterus

Advanced age

Figure 26: Reasons for choosing Caesarean section

26.6.4.2. Reasons for choosing the vaginal route

It should be noted that one or more reasons may be reported by a single patient (Figure27).

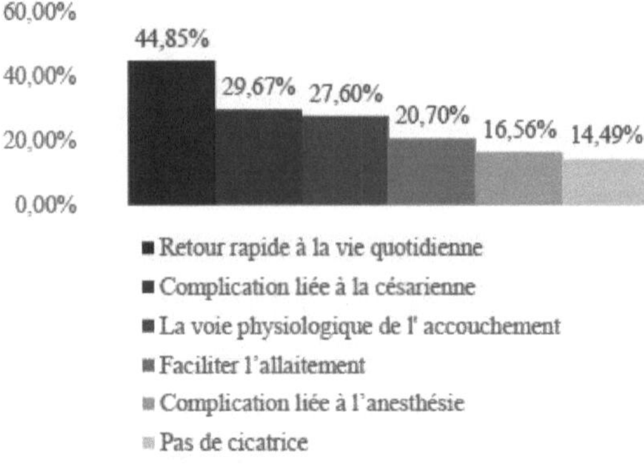

- Quick return to everyday life
- Complications associated with caesarean section
- The physiological way of childbirth
- Making breastfeeding easier
- Complications associated with anaesthesia
- No scarring

Figure 27: Reasons for choosing the vaginal route

27.7. Overall assessment of fear of childbirth

Total fear of childbirth scores ranged from 21 to 84, with a mean of 53.53 and a standard deviation of 13.7.

The averages for the five LFS factors are summarised in Table VI.

Table VI: Assessment of fear of childbirth

	Average (SD)	Minimum	Maximum
Anticipating a Trauma	12,75(±3)	4	16
Cognitive intrusion	11,93(±4,72)	5	20
Avoidance	7,47(±3,04)	3	10
Emotional loss	7,06(±3,22)	4	16
Hyperstimulation	14,32(±4,4)	5	20
Total EPA score	53,53(±13,78)	21	84

SD: Standard deviation, EPA: Fear of Childbirth Scale

2. ANALYTICAL STUDY

2.1. Factors associated with fear of childbirth

2.1.1. Socio-demographic factors

The only socio-demographic factor statistically significantly associated with fear of childbirth was low socioeconomic status **(p=0.021)** (Table VII).

Table VII: Univariate study of socio-demographic factors associated with fear of childbirth fear of childbirth

\ Variables	Mod .л lity	Averages EPA	Ec art-standard	Minimum	Mr.iiiinuin	P-valear
_A 2ï	<30 years	52 ;9	14.38	21	84	P=0.321
	>30йП5	55	12,29	27	75	
Situation	C elib atary	54	11.84	33	66	P=0.93

mairi пнжЫ	Manee	53,52	13.86	21	84	P=0.527
Profession	Woman at home	53.84	13.79	21	84	
	Other	52.31	13.84	25	84	
Socio-economic level	Top	5133	8.5	45	61	**P=0,021**
	M oyen	52.51	13.38	21	84	
	Low	60,5	15.17	30	84	
Study level	Pnniaire	54.27	15.86	21	84	P=0.2U
	Secondane	54.93	12.85	24	84	
	University	50,96	12.68	29	84	
Socio-deinograpic origin	Rural	54,065	13.12	21	84	P=0,671
	Uabaine	53.20	14,21	23	84	

EPA: Fear of childbirth scale

2.1.2. Factors linked to events and lifestyle

The analytical study showed no lifestyle factors significantly associated with fear of childbirth (table VIII).

Table VIII: Univariate analysis of event-related and lifestyle factors associated with fear of childbirth

Variables	Modality	Averages EPA	Standard deviation	Minimum	Maximum	P- value
Recent bereavement	Yes	57,066	17	21	84	P=0,303
	No	53,24	13,50	23	84	
Sports activities	Yes	54,14	12,062	34	84	P=0,804
	No	53,43	14,065	21	84	

EPA: Fear of childbirth scale

2.1.3. Gynaeco-obstetrical history:

The analytical study did not show any factor linked to previous pregnancies to be significantly associated with fear of childbirth (table IX).

Table IX: Univariate study of factors related to previous pregnancies associated with fear of childbirth

fear of childbirth

Variables	Modality	Averages EPA	Standard deviation	Minimum	Maximum	P- value
Repeated abortions	Yes	53,77	10,61	30	70	P=0,38
	No	52,96	14,34	21	84	
Recourse episiotomy	Yes	53,49	14,05	23	84	P=0,126
	No	49,46	12,35	29	84	
Information before episiotomy	Yes	50,5	12,62	26	74	P=0,712
	No	51,57	13,26	23	84	
Negative experiences of childbirth	Yes	52,67	13,6	23	84	P=0,166
	No	48,51	12,39	29	84	

2.1.4. Data relating to the current pregnancy :

For the current pregnancy, the factor statistically significantly associated with fear of childbirth was primiparity ($p = 0.001$). (Table X)

Table X: Univariate study of factors related to current pregnancy associated with fear of

childbirth

of childbirth

Variable	Modality	Averages EPA	Standard deviation	Minimum	Maximum	P-value
Primiparity	Yes	61,01	12,88	35	84	**P=0,001**
	No	52,96	13,76	25	84	
Gestational age	2nd quarter	56,79	13,95	31	84	P=0,60
	3rd quarter	52,50	13,61	21	84	
Infertility/AIDS	Pregnancy induced	54,35	9,91	36	72	P=0,80
	Spontaneous pregnancy	53,45	14,11	21	84	
Planned nature of pregnancy	Yes	53,21	13,95	21	84	P=0,618
	No	54,28	13,44	25	84	
Follow-up pregnancy	Well monitored	52,93	13,73	21	84	P=0,202
	No follow-up	56,105	13,89	27	84	
Desired character of the baby's sex	Désiré	52,01	12,47	21	77	P=0 ,214
	Neutral	55,61	14,52	25	84	
	Unwanted	54,64	17,95	27	84	
Pathology during pregnancy	Yes	51,94	12,97	24	84	P=0,273
	No	53,58	14,29	21	84	
	Not screened	58,46	11,14	39	75	

EPA: Fear of childbirth scale

2.1.5. Women's knowledge of childbirth :

Factors related to women's knowledge of childbirth and statistically significantly associated with fear of childbirth were (Table XI):

- Information received from forums and social networks (p=0.038).
- Knowledge about epidurals (p=0.015).

Table XI: The univariate study of factors related to women's knowledge associated with fear of childbirth

Variables	Modality	Average EPA	Standard deviation	Minimum	Maximum	P-value
Information received Forums and Social networks	Yes	53,18	13,73	21	84	**P=0,038**
	No	65	10,93	52	84	
Information received from doctors and midwives	Yes	55	14,39	23	84	P=0,230
	No	52,59	13,36	21	84	
The sources concern for the woman	Women's health	51,58	15,14	21	84	P=0,488
	Baby's health	54,55	13,07	25	84	
	The work	54,22	14,09	21	84	P=0,065
	The birth itself	53,20	13,65	23	84	
	Post-partum	47 ,47	11,12	27	66	
Knowledge of preparation for birth and parenthood	Yes	52,1	12,37	25	84	P=0,252
	No	54,41	14,56	21	84	
Knowledge about	Yes	51,46	12,97	25	84	**P=0,015**

epidurals	No	56,21	14,41	21	84	
Knowledge of how to manage of pain	Yes	53,90	13,95	30	84	P=0,407
	No	5,80	13,01	21	84	

2.2. The association between EPA and the choice of delivery route

We noted a statistically significant association between a high EPA score and the choice of caesarean section as the delivery method (p<0.001). (Table XII)

Table XII: Univariate study of LFS factors associated with route of delivery of delivery

	Average EPA	Standard deviation	Minimum	Maximum	P-value
By vaginal route	48,9	11,2	23	72	**<0,001**
Caesarean section	56	14,4	21	84	

EPA: Fear of childbirth scale

2.3. Factors associated with the choice of caesarean section

2.3.1. Socio-demographic factors

The socio-demographic factor statistically significantly associated with the choice of caesarean section was low socioeconomic status (p=0.020). (Table XIII)

Table XIII: Socio-demographic factors associated with the choice of caesarean section

* Parametric chi-square test

	Odds ratio (OR)	IC95%	(P-value) * (P-value)
Age (< 30 versus > 30)	1,074	[0,855 -1,348]	0,317
Marital status (single versus married)	1,552	[1,398- 1,723]	0,76
Profession	0,444	[0,436- 1,823]	1,041
Level socio-economic (low versus medium/high)	1,351	[1,106- 1,650]	**0,020**
Level of study (primary + secondary versus university)	1,115	[0,884- 1,407]	0,213
Origin socio-demographic (urban versus rural)	1,040	[0,848 -1,276]	0,414

*Parametric chi-square test

2.3.2. Factors linked to events and lifestyle

The analytical study did not show any lifestyle factors significantly associated with the choice of caesarean section (table XIV).

Table XIII: Event and lifestyle factors associated with the choice of Caesarean section caesarean section

Variables	OR	95% CI	(P-value) * (P-value)

Recent bereavement (no versus yes)	0,736	[0,587- 0,923]	0,059
Sporting activity (no versus yes)	0,1047	[0,769- 1,425]	0,461

* Parametric test of k | hi-deux

2.3.3. Gynaecological and obstetrical history

In univariate analysis, the factors related to previous pregnancies that were statistically significantly associated with the choice of caesarean section were (Table XV):

- Use of episiotomy (p=0.001).
- Information prior to episiotomy (p=0.018).

Table XIV: Factors related to previous pregnancies associated with the choice of caesarean section

Variables	R	95% CI	(P-value) * (P-value)
Repeated abortion (yes versus no)	1,110	[0,884- 1,394]	0,220
Recourse à episiotomy (yes versus no)	1,786	[1,235- 2,583]	**0,001**
Information before episiotomy (yes versus no)	1,717	[1,012- 2,913]	**0,018**
Negative experience of childbirth (yes versus no)	1,316	[0,931- 1,860]	0,112

* Parametric chi-square test

2.3.4. Data relating to the current pregnancy

For the current pregnancy, the factor statistically significantly associated with the choice of caesarean section was primiparity (p = 0.001). (Table XVI)

Table XV: Pregnancy-related factors associated with the choice of caesarean section

Variables	OR	95% CI	(P-value) * (P-value)
Primiparity (yes versus no)	1,422	[1,156- 1,749]	**0,001**
Gestational age (13-32SA versus >33)	1,110	[0,893- 1,380]	0,238
Infertility/PMA (yes versus no)	0,920	[0,703- 1,203]	0,367
Planned nature of pregnancy (yes versus no)	1,089	[0,883- 1,343]	0,274
Well-followed character of the pregnancy (good follow-up versus poor follow-up)	0,825	[0,667- 1,021]	0,083
Desired character of the baby's sex (unwanted	0,794	[0,501- 1,258]	0,190

versus wanted/neutral)			
Pathology during pregnancy (yes versus no)	0,885	[0,640- 1,222]	0,361

PMA: medically assisted procreation /*: parametric chi-square test

2.3.5. Women's knowledge of childbirth

The analytical study did not show any factor related to women's knowledge to be significantly associated with the choice of caesarean section (Table XVII).

Table XVI: Factors related to women's knowledge associated with the choice of Caesarean section

caesarean section

Variables	OR	IC95%	(P-value) * (P-value)
Information received forums and social networks (yes versus no)	0,982	[0,553- 1,745]	0,659
Information received from doctor and midwife (yes versus no)	1,030	[0,839- 1,263]	0,452
Preparation for birth and parenthood (yes versus no)	1,060	[0,858- 1,310]	0,346
Epidural (yes versus no)	1,098	[0,889- 1,341]	0,226
Reduction in pain (yes versus no)	1,031	[0,788- 1,349]	0,482

* Parametric chi-square test

4 DISCUSSION

The results obtained were analysed taking into account the previous work mentioned in this chapter of the scientific literature.

The aims of our study were to describe women's knowledge of vaginal delivery, to describe the level of fear of vaginal delivery (using the EPA fear of childbirth scale) and to explore the factors associated with avoidance of vaginal delivery.

This chapter then discusses the strengths and weaknesses of the study. Recommendations and a conclusion are given in the final section.

1. CHARACTERISTICS OF PARTICIPANTS

Our sample consisted of 200 participants. We were unable to reach 380 participants due to time constraints. The average age of the women was 28.3 years, with a standard deviation of 5.7. Of the women, 97% were married, while 62% came from urban areas. 69.5% of the women had no more than secondary education. Almost half of the participants were housewives.

The participants were women who were in their 2nd or 3rd trimester of pregnancy and had no complications leading to a high-risk pregnancy or communication difficulties.

2. THE CHOICE OF DELIVERY METHOD

In our sample (n=200), 65.5% of women surveyed preferred to give birth by caesarean section. This preference is mainly influenced by various medical factors, including obstetric and neonatal trauma, labour abnormalities, instrumental deliveries and episiotomies. Other reasons include fear of childbirth (tocophobia) and being primiparous. Fear of post-partum complications, such as incontinence and repercussions on sex life, also contribute to this choice.

In addition, the study by M. Chabbert and J. Wendland concerned the impact of fear of childbirth on the mode of delivery and post-traumatic stress in women in 2016. This research explored how fear of childbirth could influence birth canal preferences and lead to post-traumatic stress disorders in the post-partum period (Chabbert & Wendland, 2016).

In our study, the remaining 34.5% of women surveyed opted for vaginal delivery. These women were motivated by physiological reasons such as a rapid return to daily life, the natural physiology of childbirth, the facilitation of breastfeeding, as well as concerns related to the potential complications of caesarean section, in particular complications related to anaesthesia and aesthetic aspects.

Similarly, a French study carried out in 2020 into childbirth practices found that natural childbirth protects the woman and the newborn from a number of complications (Dick-Read, 2020)

3. FEAR OF CHILDBIRTH

To measure fear of childbirth, we used a valid scale (EPA). In fact, this scale has been used by several authors, in addition to the study that was used for its psychometric validation (Masson, 2012).

The average LFS score in our sample was 53.53 points, with a minimum score of 21 and a maximum of 84. The results indicated that the twenty-one items making up the LFS were related.

In our study, we found that the mean EPA score obtained by all the women included (n=200) was 53.53, with a standard deviation of 13.7 [21-84]. This result was consistent with that found in the study by Béland et al. who adapted and validated this scale in French (Masson,

2012).

The sub-scores obtained for the five dimensions of fear of childbirth, with averages between 7.06 and 14.32, were also comparable to those obtained in the study cited above. The first dimension (anticipation of a traumatic birth) had a score between 4 and 16 with a mean of 12.75(±3). The second dimension (cognitive instruction) had a score between 5 and 20 with an average of 11.93(±4.72). The third dimension (avoidance) had a score between 3 and 10 with a mean of 7.47(±3.04). The fourth dimension (emotional blunting) had a score between 4 and 16 with a mean of 7.06(±3.22). The fifth dimension (hyperstimulation) had a score between 5 and 20 with an average of 14.32(±4.4).

Scores were calculated by adding together the scores for the different items in each dimension, with a high score indicating significant fear.

Leclerc's 2016 study found an average of 8.5 for anticipation of a traumatic birth with an associated standard deviation of 2.5 (score between 4 and 16); 7.4 for cognitive intrusion with an associated standard deviation of 3.3 (score between 5 and 20); 4.2 for avoidance with an associated standard deviation of 2.0 (score between 3 and 12); 5.4 for emotional blunting with an associated standard deviation of 2.1 (score between 4 and 16) and 10.6 for hyperstimulation with an associated standard deviation of 3.5 (score between 5 and 20) (Leclerc, 1993).

4. THE RELATIONSHIP BETWEEN FEAR OF CHILDBIRTH AND THE CHOICE OF CESAREAN SECTION

In our study, we found that fear of childbirth and the choice of caesarean section as a mode of delivery were significantly associated (p=<0.001). Several factors may contribute to this fear, including fear of the intense pain associated with vaginal birth, anxiety about potential complications during labour, or previous traumatic experiences.

Similarly, in a 2016 study by Marine Leclerc, fear of childbirth influenced the choice of delivery method (Leclerc, 1993)

However, research published in the Journal of Psychology, Obstetrics and Gynaecology in 2017, was conducted by Ryding et al the study had shown that there was no significant association between tocophobia and caesarean section rates (Ryding et al., 2015).

In addition, a meta-analysis published in the same journal in 2018 by Räisänen et al. also reported these findings (Räisänen et al., 2013).

5. FACTORS ASSOCIATED WITH FEAR AND CHOICE OF CHILDBIRTH

5.1. Tocophobia

Fear of pain or tocophobia was one of the most common reasons why women might choose a caesarean section. In our study, tocophobia was present in 90 women. This was similar to Tournier's study presented in 2023 looking at fear of childbirth in France (Staraci et al., 2012) and Dimassi's study in Tunisia et al which found a strong relationship between fear of pain and the choice of caesarean section (Dimassi et al., 2021).

The idea of intense and prolonged pain during childbirth could be very distressing for some women. They may fear that they will not be able to cope with the pain, especially if they have heard stories of difficult births from other women. The prospect of pain could be so intimidating that some women preferred a caesarean section to avoid the experience.

5.2. Obstetric and neonatal trauma

Women may also fear the potential complications associated with vaginal birth. In our study, this was noted in 93 women. Although most births would be uncomplicated, there is always a risk of complications that women might fear such as perineal tears, emergency medical interventions such as episiotomy, reported in 62 women, or health problems for the baby reported in 82 women. For some women, these perceived risks could be a source of anxiety and lead them to choose a caesarean section as a perceived safer option (Halscott et al., 2015; Jiang et al., 2017).

These results suggest that fear of childbirth may affect pregnant women's decisions about the mode of delivery and their propensity to opt for a caesarean section to avoid potential obstetric and neonatal trauma.

In addition, a study published in Acta Obstétrical et Gynécologie Scandinavica in 2015, had examined women's preferences regarding their birthing experience (Pirnat et al., 2019).

6. SOCIO-DEMOGRAPHIC FACTORS

6.1. Age

The mean age in our study was 28.3 (5.7) [18-44 years]. Age was not significantly associated with either fear of childbirth or choice of delivery method (p=0.321). Similarly, Dimassi et al, in their study carried out in the Tunis maternity hospital in 2021, did not find a statistically significant relationship between age and either fear of childbirth or the chosen mode of delivery (Dimassi et al., 2021). Also, this result was supported in the literature by several studies which suggested that fear and the choice of childbirth are not influenced by age but that this fear could be correlated to the psychology of the woman.

Another retrospective analysis by Hannah G. Dahlen and Anderson in 2018 of medical records examined the relationship between maternal age and choice of caesarean section in a given population and found no significant correlation (Dahlen et al., 2013).

In contrast, a 2015 Chinese study reported a relationship between young age and fear of childbirth (Gao et al., 2015).

Age may play a role in how women perceive and experience fear of childbirth, although this may vary from person to person. Age can be linked to fear of childbirth in a number of ways. Younger women may experience additional anxiety due to their lack of experience and knowledge of pregnancy, childbirth and motherhood. For this reason, the study by Chen et al in 2020 showed a significant association between young maternal age and fear of childbirth, which could lead to an increased likelihood of caesarean section (da Silva et al., 2003).

6.2. Marital status

In our study, the vast majority of women were married (97%), which is explained by the low number of pregnancies outside marriage in our society.

Marital status, in our series, was not significantly related to choice of route of delivery (p=0.76). This result is similar to that of the study by Garcia P et al in 2018 who showed that there was no significant difference in the choice of caesarean section between married and unmarried women. These results challenge preconceived notions that married women may prefer caesarean section over unmarried women (Pirnat et al., 2019).

In contrast, according to a study conducted in six European countries, married Norwegian women were protected from fear of childbirth (Ferreira et al., 2015).

It is unlikely that marital status in itself has a direct impact on the choice to use a caesarean section as the results of the study by Smith K, et al in 2023 showed that married women tended to report lower levels of fear of childbirth than single or unmarried women. However, some aspects of marital status may influence decisions about childbirth ("Editorial", 2009).

6.3. Professional situation

Our study showed that occupation did not influence the choice of caesarean section and fear of childbirth, but the majority of our participants were housewives (79.5%). Similarly, Tania bosshart and Julie pugin, in their study conducted in 2021, found no statistically significant correlation between occupational status and fear of childbirth, nor between occupational status and the mode of childbirth chosen (Tania & Julie, 2021).

In contradiction with our results, a study conducted in Marseille in 2020 by S. Riquet, the main objective of which was to evaluate fear in pregnant women, showed that professional situation had a significant correlation (p=0.027) with fear of childbirth. This could be explained by the fact that work-related stress can influence the choice of childbirth route (Riquet et al., 2020).

Similarly, in a study conducted in Tunisia by Dimassi et al looking at the free choice of caesarean section, professional status was significantly associated with this choice (Dimassi et al., 2021).

6.4. Level of study

In our series, level of education was not significantly associated either with fear of childbirth or with the choice of caesarean section (p=0.213). Our result is similar to that of the study by Dimassi et al, who found that higher education level did not influence the choice of caesarean section (Dimassi et al., 2021).

However, the level of education could play a role in the choice of caesarean section, although this may vary according to several factors, including medical knowledge, cultural beliefs, personal concerns and healthcare practices in a region. Furthermore, S. Riquet et al. in their study showed that the level of education was significantly related to the choice of caesarean section (p=0.03)[3].

6.5. Socio-economic level

In our study, we found that the association between socio-economic level and the choice of caesarean section and fear of childbirth was significantly negative (p=0.020). In fact, the highest mean scores for fear were recorded in women with a low socio-economic level (mean score of 60 versus a mean EPA score of 52 for women with a high socio-economic level). The level of fear was 1.3 times higher in women from low socio-economic backgrounds. This could be due to unfavourable living conditions and lack of access to care and information for poor people, whereas women from wealthier backgrounds had easier access to information. Thus, the relationship between socio-economic level and fear of childbirth highlights persistent inequalities in access to maternal health care and underscores the need for policies and programmes aimed at reducing these disparities.

In the same vein, this link was proven by another Indian study conducted by Anita et al in 2019 where the level of fear of childbirth was more than 2 times higher in women belonging to a low socioeconomic level (OR=2.804, 95% CI [1.296 - 6.068], (P=0.009) (Nath et al., 2019).

7. GYNAECO-OBSTETRIC ANTECEDENTS

7.1. Parity

Several studies have looked at the fear of childbirth and the factors that trigger this fear.

Primiparity refers to giving birth for the first time. It's an exciting time, but one that's also often filled with anxiety and fear, especially when it comes to giving birth. Many women feel apprehensive about giving birth, as it is an unknown event and is often described as painful.

In our study, we found that primiparity influenced the level of fear and the choice of mode of delivery. Primiparous women were 1.4 times more likely to develop a high level of fear and to choose caesarean section than multiparous women (OR=1.422, 95% CI [1.156- 1.749], **(P=0.001).** The mean EPA score in primiparous women was higher (61.01). This finding could be explained by the lack of experience and by the fact that the phenomenon of vaginal delivery was unknown and dismal for primiparous women. It was therefore associated with an increased risk of caesarean section, partly due to the uncertainty and anxiety associated with vaginal birth. In addition, fear of childbirth, also known as tocophobia, can be a determining factor in the decision to opt for a caesarean section. Primiparity was a risk factor for fear in some studies. In fact, the study conducted by Lucie Tournier in 2020 looking at the factors influencing attempted vaginal delivery found a significant link between primiparity, the choice of Caesarean section and fear of childbirth (Staraci et al., 2012).

However, another Tunisian study conducted in 2020 by Dimessi et al did not find a significant link (p=0.38) (Dimassi et al., 2021).

In our study, some women had opted for a planned caesarean section in their first pregnancy for medical reasons such as a history of serious complications during childbirth. Others chose an elective caesarean section for personal reasons, such as fear of vaginal delivery or a preference for planned birth.

7.2. History of abortion

In our study, a history of abortion was not significantly associated with fear of childbirth or the choice of caesarean section as a mode of delivery. However, the percentage of women with repeat abortions was only 8%.

Some women may have had an intense fear of the vaginal route due to previous abortion experience. This fear may be linked to previous emotional or physical trauma, negative perceptions of the vaginal route, apprehensions about pain or other factors. Indeed, a study conducted by Lok et al in 2019 showed a very strong link between a history of repeated abortions and the choice of caesarean section for subsequent pregnancies (Ney et al., 1994).

8. DATA RELATING TO EVENTS AND LIFESTYLE

8.1. Recent bereavement

The recent bereavement may have intensified the fear of childbirth in some pregnant women. However, it can have a profound emotional impact on a pregnant woman and influence her decision regarding the mode of delivery, including the choice of a caesarean section. In our study, we investigated the relationship between recent bereavement and fear of childbirth on the one hand and the choice of caesarean section on the other. This relationship was not significant with fear of childbirth (p=0.303) or with the choice of caesarean section (p=0.059). This contradicted a study conducted in six European countries in 2015 by Ryding et al. (Ryding et al., 2015) and this result may be explained by the fact that the number of women who had experienced a recent bereavement did not exceed 15 out of 200, i.e. a percentage of 8%.

8.2. Sporting activity

Several studies suggest that sporting activity during pregnancy can play an important role in reducing fear of childbirth and could have positive effects on maternal and neonatal outcomes.

In our study, no more than 13.5% of women took part in sporting activities. We did not find a significant relationship between sporting activity and fear of childbirth or choice of childbirth.

In contrast, a Norwegian study in 2018 by Hakstad et al examined the relationship between physical activity and fear of childbirth in pregnant women, and showed a significantly positive link $p<0.001$ (Haakstad et al., 2018).

Another study carried out by Parla Clara Santous et al in 2016 on a sample of Portuguese women showed that sporting activity helped women to overcome their fear of childbirth and vaginal delivery (Santos et al., 2016).

9. DATA ON PREVIOUS BIRTHS

9.1. Episiotomy

In our study, episiotomy was significantly associated (p= 0.001) with the choice of caesarean section. Episiotomy is a surgical incision made in the perineum to widen the passage of the baby during childbirth, and can be experienced negatively by women. This finding could explain the fear of childbirth and the decision to request a caesarean section in the face of the desire to avoid an episiotomy. Similarly, in a 2015 study by Halscott TL et al looking at episiotomy and caesarean section, the Techniques and Complications results found that episiotomy increased fear of childbirth and led women to choose a caesarean section of convenience (Halscott et al., 2015).

On the other hand, another study carried out in 2012 by Haines et al investigating the selective or systematic use of episiotomy for vaginal delivery showed that there was no significant link between episiotomy and the choice of caesarean section as a mode of delivery (Haines et al., 2012).

9.2. Negative experiences of childbirth

In our study, the negative experience of childbirth was not significantly related to the choice of caesarean section (p=0.112). In addition, several studies found no significant correlation between the negative experience of childbirth and the choice of Caesarean section. For example, a meta-analysis by O'connell et al in 2017 examined this relationship and concluded that there was no significant association between postpartum psychological trauma and subsequent choice of caesarean section (O'connell et al., 2017).

Thus, although the experience of childbirth may have an impact on the preferences of pregnant women, it seems that this factor is not always significantly associated with the choice of caesarean section (Haines et al., 2012).

However, in other studies, previous childbirth experiences, whether personal or those of close relatives, may influence the choice of a caesarean section. If a woman has had a difficult or traumatic birth in the past, she may fear reliving the same experience and choose a caesarean section as a perceived less stressful alternative. This was described in the study by Srinivas et al. which showed the relationship between negative experience of childbirth and preference for Caesarean section in young women prior to childbirth (Srinivas et al., 2010).

10. DATA RELATING TO THIS PREGNANCY

10.1. Gestational age

In general, pregnant women react differently to the approach of childbirth. Some may experience increased anxiety rather than positive excitement. This reaction can be explained by the accentuation of physical changes during the final months of pregnancy, as well as concerns about childbirth and motherhood. What's more, the fear of childbirth can intensify as the date approaches. This was demonstrated in a study conducted by S. Riquet et al, who found that the fear of childbirth score increased from one trimester to the next, peaking in the 3rd trimester (57.5%) with a significantly positive association (p=0.02) (Riquet et al., 2020).

Gestational age at the time of our questionnaire was between 16 and 41 weeks of amenorrhoea. However, it was not significantly associated either with fear of childbirth (p=0.60) or with the choice of caesarean section in the present study (p=0.238).

The length of pregnancy (in weeks) does not have a major or determining impact on the decision to have a caesarean section, given the existence of other influencing factors such as the mother's health, the baby's position, specific medical complications or obstetric history, which play a much more important role in this decision.

10.2. Monitoring pregnancy

Pregnancy monitoring played a crucial role in the relationship with fear of childbirth. Attentive and caring monitoring could help to reduce anxiety and fears about childbirth by offering emotional support, accurate information and establishing a relationship of trust between the pregnant woman and the healthcare professionals.

In 2016, Ghadeer et al found a significant link between good pregnancy monitoring and a reduction in fear of childbirth (Al Ghadeer et al., 2021).

This was not consistent with our study. Although 81% of the women had followed their pregnancies well, the scores for fear of childbirth were high and there was no significant link between follow-up and fear or the mode chosen with (p= 0.202). This nuance could call into question antenatal care. For this reason, it is very important to organise education sessions on the physiology of childbirth. On the one hand, these sessions contribute to an understanding of what happens in the body during childbirth and can considerably reduce anxiety and fear in pregnant women. On the other hand, they provide greater knowledge and enable expectant mothers to feel more in control of their childbirth, helping them to make informed decisions. In addition, women can learn about the different stages of childbirth and techniques for managing pain, which can prepare them to face the physical and emotional challenges. Alternatively, better-informed women are often better able to recognise the signs of potential complications, which can lead to faster and more appropriate interventions.

These sessions also help to create support networks among pregnant women, partners and families.

10.3. Problems of infertility or medically assisted procreation

Infertility and recourse to medically assisted procreation (MAP) can be difficult journeys for many couples, and the fear of childbirth could be an additional concern in this context.

Infertility can cause significant emotional stress, which can be exacerbated by fear of childbirth. Couples may fear that, having overcome infertility, the birth will not go as planned.

Indeed, a Malawian study investigating factors associated with fear of childbirth conducted by Gabrielle et al in 2017 found that fear of childbirth among women in Malawi may also be relevant to women with a history of infertility and MAP (Gabrielle et al, 2017).

However, in our study the relationship between fear of vaginal delivery and induced pregnancy was not significant (p=0.367), but women with induced pregnancy had higher fear scores than those with spontaneous pregnancy.

11. WOMEN'S KNOWLEDGE OF HOW TO GIVE BIRTH

11.1. Information sources

11.1.1. Doctor and midwife

It is important that the information received about childbirth comes from reliable, evidence-based sources. Health professionals, including doctors, midwives and mental health counsellors, could provide accurate and reassuring information to help women better understand the birthing process and reduce their fears.

In our study, the subject of childbirth was discussed by 59% of women. Only 39% of women had received information from their doctor or midwife, while the rest, especially primiparous women, had no idea what childbirth was like or had preconceived ideas about childbirth, which could have heightened their fears. We found that reliable information from the doctor and midwife had no significant effect either on fear of childbirth (p=0.230) or on the choice of

caesarean section (p=0.452).
On the other hand, several studies found that the acquisition of antenatal education by healthcare professionals had a positive impact on satisfaction and the reduction of fear of childbirth, such as the French study conducted in 2018 by Garance Cuenin studying the educational approach during pregnancy (Cuenin, 2018).

11.1.2. Friends and family, social media, forum

False information could have a significant impact on the fear of childbirth, as it could amplify pregnant women's fears and anxieties.
A Quebec study conducted by Raymonde Gagnon in 2017 showed that the influence of information obtained from friends and family on fear of childbirth could be significant. The information, experiences and opinions shared by family, friends or other relatives could influence a pregnant woman's perceptions and fears of childbirth, since they only shared their negative experiences and fears of childbirth. The same was true of social networks and the media (Gagnon, 2017).
On the other hand, another study in Saudi Arabia by Ghadaar et al, looking at the impact of social networks on pregnant women, found that social networks and the Internet increased women's knowledge of the birthing process and reduced their fear of childbirth (Al Ghadeer et al., 2021).
This was consistent with our study, which found a significantly positive relationship between sources of information from family and friends, the media and fear of vaginal delivery (p=0.038).
It was essential for pregnant women to seek information from reliable sources, such as health professionals, reputable medical books and trusted websites, to obtain accurate information about childbirth and thus reduce the fear associated with this process.

11.2. Preparing for birth and parenthood

Preparing for birth and parenthood is an important process for future parents. It generally includes courses and information sessions aimed at preparing parents for childbirth and the first days with their baby.
In our study, none of the women had attended a PNP course and 38% of the women who knew about preparation for childbirth and parenthood through social networks were unaware of its importance and impact on maternal relief and well-being.
A number of studies have been carried out on PNP, and all the results show that preparation for birth and parenthood has an effect on women's physical and mental health. These courses provide information on the birthing process, different pain management options, breathing and relaxation techniques, as well as advice on labour and birth. This can take away negative feelings and worries. Attending these PNP sessions could boost self-confidence (Cuenin, 2018).
However, in our study we found no significant relationship between knowledge of PNP and fear of childbirth (p=0.252) or choice of caesarean section (p=0.346).
Preparation for birth and parenthood can vary from country to country and culture to culture, but the main aim is to help women manage all phases of childbirth more effectively and to help couples feel informed, confident and prepared to welcome their baby and face the challenges of parenthood.

11.3. Epidural analgesia

The epidural can be a reassuring option for women who are afraid of the pain of childbirth. In Tunisia, epidural analgesia is not yet considered in public hospitals, only in private clinics

(Dimassi et al., 2021).

On the other hand, epidurals were rapidly established in Quebec, varying between 40% and 90%.

Depending on the region and the establishment. It is recognised that the epidural not only relieved pain. It also led to a cascade of interventions which have other consequences for the progress of labour and birth (Sinclair, 2018).

In our study, we found a significant link between knowledge of the epidural and fear of childbirth (p=0.015). This could be explained by the psychological relief provided by this technique.

Epidurals can indeed be an attractive option for women who have a fear of childbirth, as they offer effective pain relief while allowing the mother to remain conscious and actively participate in the birth. By reducing pain, epidurals can also help to reduce the anxiety and fear associated with childbirth (Leclerc, 1993).

On the other hand, the Gagnon Raymound study in 2017 showed that epidural failure, although rare, could occur in certain cases, particularly when analgesia was not effective in relieving the pain of labour sufficiently. In such cases, some women might be faced with the choice of a caesarean section to ensure adequate pain relief during labour. In this study, knowledge of epidurals had no effect on the choice of caesarean section (Gagnon, 2017).

It is essential that pregnant women discuss pain relief options during childbirth in detail with the medical team, including alternatives to the epidural and possible scenarios in the event of epidural failure. This discussion could help them make informed decisions about their birth plan and feel better prepared for any eventuality during labour and birth.

12. STRENGTHS AND LIMITATIONS OF THE STUDY

12.1. Highlights

A number of strengths were highlighted:

- Our research environment was the CHU Hedi Chaker Sfax. This is a level III maternity hospital which is a reference centre for scientific research. This hospital is the point of admission for different categories of pregnant women, which will contribute to the richness and generalisation of the results.
- We used a fear scale (EPA). This is a valid scale, translated into Arabic, which facilitates interpretation of the data and guarantees valid results that are comparable with the literature.
- We carried out an analytical study, which enabled us to identify hypotheses and also to check the links between the variables with a view to revealing the risk factors so that appropriate solutions could be put in place.
- Sampling was random. All eligible women had an equal opportunity to take part in the study, in order to obtain a representative sample for better generalisation of the results.

12.2. The limits

- Due to time constraints, we were unable to recruit the number of subjects required for the study. Our sample was not representative, i.e. it did not represent the general population in terms of numbers, which limits the generalisability of the results.
- Studies on fear of childbirth in Tunisia are limited.
- The Arabic version of the fear scale had not yet been validated.
- The data collection period was limited.

13. RECOMMENDATIONS

❖ Follow childbirth preparation sessions, with objectives spread over several sessions. We suggest:

J 1st session: during this session, the physiology of the female genital system is explained to the woman.
D 2(th) session: this allows us to inform the woman about the birth process.
J 3rd session: during this session, the woman is free to ask questions which are answered.

- *S* 4th session: learning how to breathe correctly.
- *S* 5th session: consisting of yoga, haptonomy and swimming to relax mums.
- *S* 6(th) session: consists of preparing the perineal muscles for childbirth.

❖ Training midwives to listen, support and advise pregnant women who are going through periods of anxiety and fear of childbirth.

❖ Including the family and friends in the educational process: promotes a dynamic, stimulating and supportive learning environment. This not only makes it possible to achieve educational objectives more effectively, but also strengthens relationships and promotes the overall well-being of women.

❖ Psychological care for women throughout pregnancy, childbirth and even the post-partum period, which is crucial to their emotional well-being and mental health.

❖ Work on access to peridurals in public hospitals: Effective pain relief, peridurals offer women an important option for managing pain during labour and birth.

❖ Avoid systematic use of instruments (episiotomy, forceps, etc.).

5 CONCLUSION

Pregnancy and childbirth are natural physiological processes, but they can also be accompanied by concerns and challenges. It is important for pregnant women to have regular medical check-ups, to find out about the various antenatal care options available and to prepare emotionally for the arrival of their baby.

We conducted this cross-sectional, descriptive and analytical study in the gynaecology-obstetrics department of the CHU Hedi Chaker in Sfax, Tunisia. The objectives of our work were to describe women's knowledge of vaginal delivery, to explore the factors associated with vaginal delivery absconding and to describe the level of fear of vaginal delivery by the EPA.

The level of fear was judged to be average, with an average score of 53.53. Caesarean section was chosen as the delivery method in 65.5% of cases.

The level of fear was higher among women who had chosen Caesarean section as their delivery method. Several risk factors were revealed, including tocophobia and the occurrence of obstetric and neonatal trauma.

In the analytical study, the factors statistically associated with fear of childbirth were low socio-economic status (p=0.021), primiparity (p=0.001), knowledge of epidural analgesia (p=0.015) and information received from family and friends, the internet and forums. The relationship between fear of childbirth and the choice of caesarean section was significant (p<0.001).

The factors statistically associated with the choice of caesarean section as a method of delivery (yes versus no) were low socio-economic status (p=0.020), recourse to episiotomy and lack of information for the patient prior to the procedure (p=0.001 and p=0.018 respectively) and primiparity (p=0.001).

Consequently, it is recommended that healthcare professionals address the subject of fear, pain and mode of delivery and include it in antenatal care. However, it should be emphasised that a larger-scale study covering both the state and private sectors is needed.

6 REFERENCES

1. Al Ghadeer, H. A., Al Kishi, N. A., Almubarak, D. M., Almurayhil, Z., Alhafith, F., Al Makainah, B. A., Algurini, K. H., Aljumah, M. M., Busaleh, M. M., Altaweel, N. A., & Alamer, M. H. (2021). Pregnancy-Related Anxiety and Impact of Social Media Among Pregnant Women Attending Primary Health Care. *Cureus.*
2. Chabbert, M., & Wendland, J. (2016). Experiences of childbirth and women's perceived sense of control during labour: An impact on early mother-baby relationships? *Revue de Médecine Périnatale*, *8*(4), 199-206.
3. Cuenin, G. (2018). *The educational process during pregnancy.*
4. Dahlen, H., Schmied, V., Dennis, C.-L., & Thornton, C. (2013). Rates of obstetric intervention during birth and selected maternal and neonatal outcomes for low risk women born in Australia compared to those born overseas. *BMC Pregnancy and Childbirth*, *13.*
5. da Silva, A. A. M., Simões, V. M. F., Barbieri, M. A., Bettiol, H., Lamy-Filho, F., Coimbra, L. C., & Alves, M. T. S. S. B. (2003). Young maternal age and preterm birth. *Paediatric and Perinatal Epidemiology*, *17*(4), 332-339.
6. Dick-Read, G. (2020, November 6). *Physiological childbirth: A natural alternative.* Daylily Paris.
7. Dimassi, K., Melki, M., Chebbi, A., & Rafrafi, R. (2021). Le libre choix de la voie d'accouchement : Enquête auprès de femmes tunisiennes. *La Tunisie Médicale*, *99*(08-09), 903-910.
8. Dumont, A., & Guilmoto, C. Z. (2020). Trop et pas assez à la fois : Le double fardeau de la césarienne: *Population & Sociétés*, *N° 581* (9), 1-4.
9. Editorial. (2009). *Journal of Psychosomatic Obstetrics & Gynecology*, *30*(2), 81-82.
10. Faten, E., Sarah, A., Rahma, D., Sana, E., & Majda, C. (2017). Evolution after the Jasmine revolution of mental disorders in Tunisia. *PSN*, *15* (2), 7-17.
11. Ferreira, C. R., Orsini, M. C., Vieira, C. R., do Amarante Paffaro, A. M., & Silva, R. R. (2015). Prevalence of anxiety symptoms and depression in the third gestational trimester. *Archives of Gynecology and Obstetrics*, *291*(5), 999-1003.
12. Gabrielle et al (2017). *Impact of women with a history of infertility and MAP on fear of childbirth.*
13. Gagnon, R. (2017). *Thesis presented for the degree of Philosophiae Doctor (Ph.D.) in Applied Humanities.*
14. Gao, L.-L., Liu, X. J., Fu, B. L., & Xie, W. (2015). Predictors of childbirth fear among pregnant Chinese women: A cross-sectional questionnaire survey. *Midwifery*, *31* (9), 865-870.
15. Haakstad, L. A. H., Vistad, I., Sagedal, L. R., Lohne-Seiler, H., & Torstveit, M. K. (2018). How does a lifestyle intervention during pregnancy influence perceived barriers to leisure-time physical activity? The Norwegian fit for delivery study, a randomized controlled trial. *BMC Pregnancy and Childbirth*, *18*, 127.
16. Haines, H. M., Rubertsson, C., Pallant, J. F., & Hildingsson, I. (2012). The influence of women's fear, attitudes and beliefs of childbirth on mode and experience of birth. *BMC Pregnancy and Childbirth*, *12*, 55.
17. Halscott, T. L., Reddy, U. M., Landy, H. J., Ramsey, P. S., Iqbal, S. N., Huang, C.-C., & Grantz, K. L. (2015). Maternal and Neonatal Outcomes by Attempted Mode of Operative Delivery From a Low Station in the Second Stage of Labor. *Obstetrics and Gynecology*, *126*(6), 1265-1272.

18. Jiang, H., Qian, X., Carroli, G., & Garner, P. (2017). Selective versus routine use of episiotomy for vaginal birth. *The Cochrane Database of Systematic Reviews*, *2*(2), CD000081.
19. Leclerc, M. (1993). *Évaluation de la peur de l'accouchement en fin de grossesse : Effet de la préparation à la naissance et à la parentalité sur celle-ci.*
20. lucie, F., & Chagno, A. (2009, de a2017). *Common fears and anxiety during pregnancy.* https://naitreetgrandir.com/fr/grossesse/sante-bien-etre/anxiete-grossesse/
21. Masson, E. (2012). *Assessment of fear of childbirth. Validation and French adaptation of a scale measuring fear of childbirth.* EM-Consulte.
https://www.em-consulte.com/article/751672/evaluation-de-la-peur-de- laccouchement-validation-
22. Nath, A., Venkatesh, S., Balan, S., Metgud, C. S., Krishna, M., & Murthy, G. V. S. (2019). The prevalence and determinants of pregnancy-related anxiety amongst pregnant women at less than 24 weeks of pregnancy in Bangalore, Southern India. *International Journal of Women's Health, 11,* 241-248.
23. Ney, P. G., Fung, T., Wickett, A. R., & Beaman-Dodd, C. (1994). The effects of pregnancy loss on women's health. *Social Science & Medicine (1982)*, *38*(9), 1193-1200.
24. O'Connell, M. A., Leahy-Warren, P., Khashan, A. S., Kenny, L. C., & O'Neill, S. M. (2017). Worldwide prevalence of tocophobia in pregnant women: Systematic review and meta-analysis. *Acta Obstetricia Et Gynecologica Scandinavica*, *96*(8), 907-920.
25. Pirnat, A., DeRoo, L. A., Skjsrven, R., & Morken, N.-H. (2019). Risk of having one lifetime pregnancy and modification by outcome of pregnancy and perinatal loss. *Acta Obstetricia et Gynecologica Scandinavica*, *98*(6), 753-760.
https://doi.org/10.1111/aogs.13534
26. Räisänen, S., Lehto, S. M., Nielsen, H. S., Gissler, M., Kramer, M. R., & Heinonen, S. (2013). Fear of childbirth predicts postpartum depression: A population-based analysis of 511,422 singleton births in Finland. *BMJ Open*, *3*(11), e004047.
27. Riquet, S., Henni, M., & Fremondiere, P. (2020). Evaluation of fear of childbirth in pregnant women. *Périnatalité*, *12*(3), 130-139.
28. Ryding, E. L., Lukasse, M., Parys, A.-S. V., Wangel, A.-M., Karro, H., Kristjansdottir, H., Schroll, A.-M., Schei, B., & Bidens Group (2015). Fear of childbirth and risk of cesarean delivery: A cohort study in six European countries. *Birth (Berkeley, Calif.)*, *42*(1), 48-55.
29. Santos, P. C., Abreu, S., Moreira, C., Santos, R., Ferreira, M., Alves, O., Moreira, P., & Mota, J. (2016). Physical Activity Patterns During Pregnancy in a Sample of Portuguese Women: A Longitudinal Prospective Study. *Iranian Red Crescent Medical Journal*, *18*(3), e22455.
30. Sinclair, I. (2018). *Psychosocial health, immigration and pregnancy outcomes.*
31. Srinivas, S. K., Fager, C., & Lorch, S. A. (2010). Evaluating Risk-Adjusted Cesarean Delivery Rate as a Measure of Obstetric Quality. *Obstetrics and gynecology*, *115*(5), 1007-1013.
32. Staraci, S., Missonnier, S., Soubieux, M.-J., & Ville, Y. (2012). Fate of a prenatal survivor in transfuser-transfused syndrome. *La psychiatrie de l'enfant*, *55*(2), 347-396.
33. Tania, B., & Julie, P. (2021). *What is the impact of caesarean section on the mother-child attachment bond?*
34. Zouaoui, B. (2021). Tunisia: 50% of births are by caesarean section, the reasons are many-Gnet news.

Appendix A
Questionnaire

We would like to ask you to answer our questionnaire as spontaneously as possible so that we can successfully complete our study. **Please note that the information and answers collected will be treated strictly anonymously.** Please tick the circle corresponding to your answer.

I. Socio-demographic data and background 1. Your age: .... 2. Your marital status: Single Married 3. Your geographical origin: Rural Urban 4. Level of education: Primary Secondary University 5. Your employment status: .... 6. Your socio-economic level: High Medium Low

7. Have you recently suffered a bereavement: No Yes 8. Your medical history: Diabetes Asthma Thrombophilia Anaemia Other

9. Your surgical history: Appendectomy Tonsillectomy EP operated Ovarian cyst operated Cholecystectomy Synechia repair Caesarean section Other: .... 10. Have you had previous miscarriages? No Yes, only 1 time Yes more than 2 times 11. Parity: ....

II. Details of your last delivery: during your last delivery 1. You gave birth: At term Before term 2. Hospital Private clinic At home 3. Did you have a foetal death in utero: No Yes

4. Did you have an episiotomy: No Yes

5. If yes, were you informed of this procedure beforehand: No Yes 6. Did you have an instrumental birth (information checked against birth records): No Yes 7. Do you have a post-partum haemorrhage (information checked with the birth records): No Yes 8. Have you had a neonatal death: No Yes 9. Did you have a retention of the last head (Information checked with the birth records): No Yes 10. Did you have an epidural: No Yes 11. Did you have a post partum complication :

No

Yes, such as infectious complications (episiotomy infection, mastitis or breast abscess) and thromboembolic complications.

III. During this pregnancy: 1. gestational age in SA: .... 2. Did you have an infertility problem : No Yes 3. Induced pregnancy : No Yes ý If yes, means of induction : ....

4. Is this pregnancy planned: No Yes 5. Regarding the current pregnancy, the number of prenatal consultations and ultrasounds: .... 6. Concerning the sex of your baby :

Not desired Desired Neutral

7. Did any somatic pathologies appear during this pregnancy?

Yes No No screened

8. Do you practise sport during this pregnancy?

No Yes

IV. Women's knowledge of childbirth: 1. Was the subject of childbirth discussed during prenatal consultations?
Yes No
If yes, by whom? Doctor Midwife 2. In addition to the information received from the doctor and/or midwife, did you receive any other information from :
Friends and family Internet, forum
Television programmes Magazines and newspapers 3. Do you worry most often about : Your health Your baby's health 4. What phase of childbirth are you most worried about?
Labour Birth proper Post partum
5. Do you know how to reduce the pain: Yes No ý If yes, how?
....

....
6. Do you know about preparation for birth and parenthood?
Yes No 7. Are you familiar with epidural analgesia? Yes No 8. If you could choose the delivery route, what would you choose?
Delivery by vaginal route Delivery by caesarean section
9. For women who chose Caesarean section: ý What are your associated factors?
Obstetric trauma Phobia about the occurrence of obstetric trauma in the newborn Instrumental delivery Tocophobia Episiotomy Abnormal labour Sexual repercussions Delivery in a uni-scarred uterus Primiparous Elderly women Incontinence problems Post-partum complications Other: ....
ý What type of anaesthetic do you prefer?
Epidural analgesia General anaesthesia Spinal anaesthesia 10. For women who have chosen to have a base birth: ý What are the advantages of natural childbirth for you?
Rapid return to everyday life Physiological aspects of childbirth Aesthetics Facilitating breastfeeding Complications related to caesarean section Complications related to anaesthesia Other: ....

Appendix B

Fear of childbirth scale :

		Not at all -1-	Rarely -2-	Sometimes -3-	Often -4-
F1 anticipation trauma	1-giving birth will be an experience Challenging				
	2-during childbirth I'm going to feel physically abused				
	3-during childbirth I will really afraid that me or my child die or be injured				
	4-during childbirth I'm going to				

	feeling anxious or horrified				
F2 intrusions Cognitive	5-thoughts and images about childbirth invade me				
	6-I have unpleasant dreams about childbirth				
	7-suddenly, I feel as if I'm in labour and I'm overcome by a feeling of fear Intense				
	8-whatever reminds me of childbirth triggers a reaction in me. intense psychological distress				
	9-which reminds me of childbirth has given me a new physical distress				
F3 avoidance	10-I try to avoid thoughts, emotions and emotions and conversations that might make me think of childbirth				
	11-I try to avoid activities and places or people that might remind me of childbirth				
	12-I find it difficult to imagine important stages in childbirth				
F4 blunting	13- I've lost interest in				
	activities I enjoy before pregnancy				
	14-I feel cut off or isolated from Other				
	15-my ability to love or to be affection is reduced				
	16-I feel that my future does not have more meaning				
F5 Hyperstimulation	17-I find it hard to fall asleep or I don't feel well. wakes me up at night				
	18-I can suddenly feel very Irritated or angry without				

	reason				
	19-I have difficulty concentrating				
	20-I always feel tense and on edge. on the alert				
	21-I react strongly to unexpected events				

Appendix C

غالبا	أحيانا	نادرا	لا		
				ستكون الولاده تجربه شاقة	F1
				اثناء الوالده سوف أشعر بالإيذاء الجسدي	
				أثناء الوالده، ا موتي أو إصابة طفلي	
				أثناء الوالده سأشعر بالقلق أو الرعب	
				الافكار والصور غير السارة عن الولاده تأتي فوقي	F2
				لدي أحلام غير سارة بشأن الوالده	
				فجأة أشعر كما لو أن المخاض في تقدم وأنني غارق في الشعور بالخوف الشديد	
				ما يذكرني بالوالده يسبب لي ضائقة نفسية شديدة	
				ما يذكرني بالوالده يسبب لي ضائقة جسدية	
				أحاول تجنب الأفكار والمشاعر والأحاديث التي قد تذكرني بالوالده	F3
				أحاول تجنب الأنشطة أو الأماكن أو الأشخاص الذين قد يذكرونني بالوالده	
				أجد صعوبة في تخيل مراحل مهمة من الوالده	

F4	فقدت اهتمامي بالأنشطة التي كنت أستمتع بها قبل الحمل				
	أشعر بالعزلة أو الانعزال عن الآخرين				
	تقل قدرتي على الحب أو أن أكون حنونًا				
	لدي شعور بأن مستقبلي ليس له معنى				
F5	أجد صعوبة في النوم أو أستيقظ في الليل				
	قد أشعر فجأة بالغضب الشديد أو الغضب دون سبب				
	أجد صعوبة في التركيز				
	أشعر دائما بالتوتر والقلق				
	أتفاعل بقوة مع الأحداث غير المتوقعة				

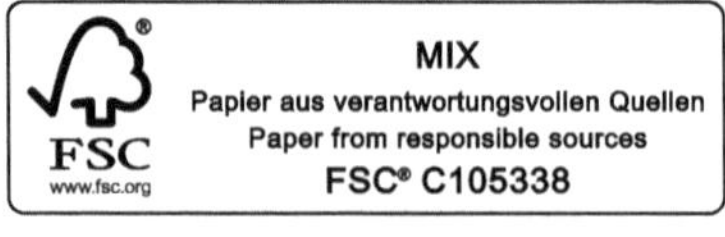

Printed by Books on Demand GmbH, Norderstedt / Germany